2016

Choosing a Medigap Policy:

A Guide to Health Insurance for People with Medicare

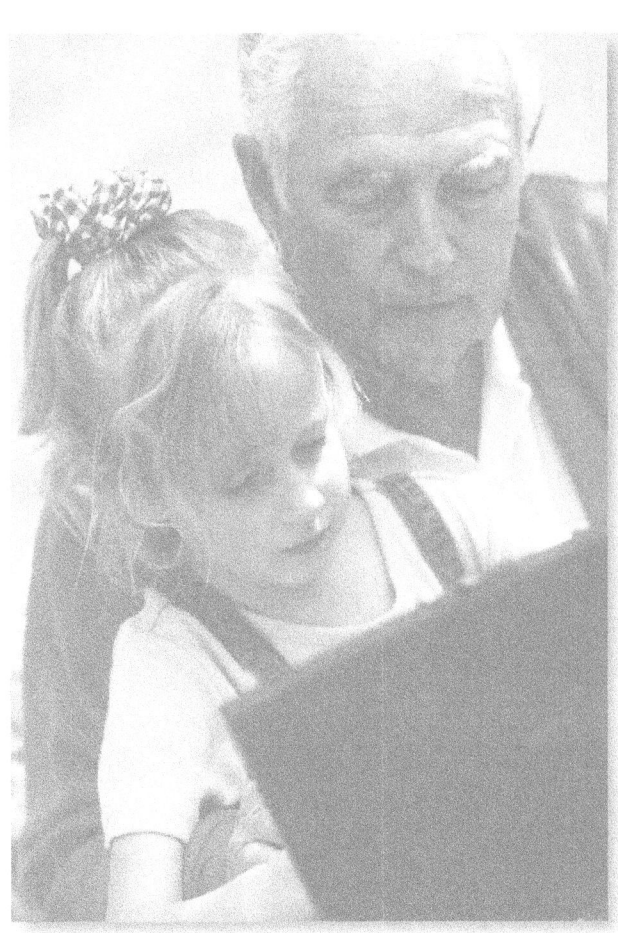

This official government guide has important information about:

- Medicare Supplement Insurance (Medigap) policies

- What Medigap policies cover

- Your rights to buy a Medigap policy

- How to buy a Medigap policy

This guide can help if you're thinking about buying a Medigap policy or already have one.

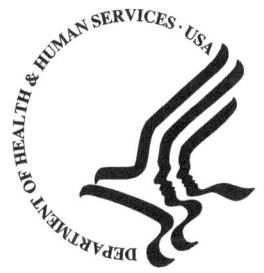

Developed jointly by the Centers for Medicare & Medicaid Services (CMS) and the National Association of Insurance Commissioners (NAIC)

Who should read this guide?

This guide helps people with Medicare understand Medicare Supplement Insurance policies (also called Medigap policies). A Medigap policy is a type of private insurance that helps you pay for some of the costs that Original Medicare doesn't cover.

Important information about this guide

The information in this booklet describes the Medicare program at the time this booklet was printed. Changes may occur after printing. Visit Medicare.gov, or call 1-800-MEDICARE (1-800-633-4227) to get the most current information. TTY users should call 1-877-486-2048.

The "2016 Choosing a Medigap Policy: A Guide to Health Insurance for People with Medicare" isn't a legal document. Official Medicare Program legal guidance is contained in the relevant statutes, regulations, and rulings.

SECTION

Medicare Basics

A brief look at Medicare

A Medicare Supplement Insurance (Medigap) Policy is a health insurance sold by private insurance companies which can help pay some of the health care costs that Original Medicare doesn't cover, like coinsurance, copayments, or deductibles. Some Medigap policies also cover certain benefits Original Medicare doesn't cover like emergency foreign travel expenses. Medigap policies don't cover your share of the costs under other types of health coverage, including Medicare Advantage Plans (like HMOs or PPOs), stand-alone Medicare Prescription Drug Plans, employer/union group health coverage, Medicaid, or TRICARE. Insurance companies generally can't sell you a Medigap policy if you have coverage through Medicaid or a Medicare Advantage Plan.

Before you learn more about Medigap policies, the next few pages provide a brief look at Medicare. If you already know the basics about Medicare and only want to learn about Medigap, skip to page 9.

Words in blue are defined on pages 49–50.

What's Medicare?

Medicare is health insurance for:

- People 65 or older
- People under 65 with certain disabilities
- People of any age with End-Stage Renal Disease (ESRD) (permanent kidney failure requiring dialysis or a kidney transplant)

The different parts of Medicare

The different parts of Medicare help cover specific services:

Medicare Part A (Hospital Insurance) helps cover

- Inpatient care in hospitals
- Skilled nursing facility, hospice, and home health care

Medicare Part B (Medical Insurance) helps cover

- Services from doctors and other health care providers, hospital outpatient care, durable medical equipment, and home health care
- Preventive services to help maintain your health and to keep certain illnesses from getting worse

Medicare Part C (Medicare Advantage)

- Includes all benefits and services covered under Part A and Part B
- Run by Medicare-approved private insurance companies
- Usually includes Medicare prescription drug coverage (Part D) as part of the plan
- May include extra benefits and services for an extra cost

Medicare Part D (Medicare Prescription Drug Coverage)

- Helps cover the cost of outpatient prescription drugs
- Run by Medicare-approved private insurance companies
- May help lower your prescription drug costs and help protect against higher costs in the future

Your Medicare coverage choices at a glance

There are 2 main ways to get your Medicare coverage — Original Medicare or a Medicare Advantage Plan. Use these steps to help you decide which way to get your coverage. See page 35 for information about Medicare Advantage Plans and Medigap policies.

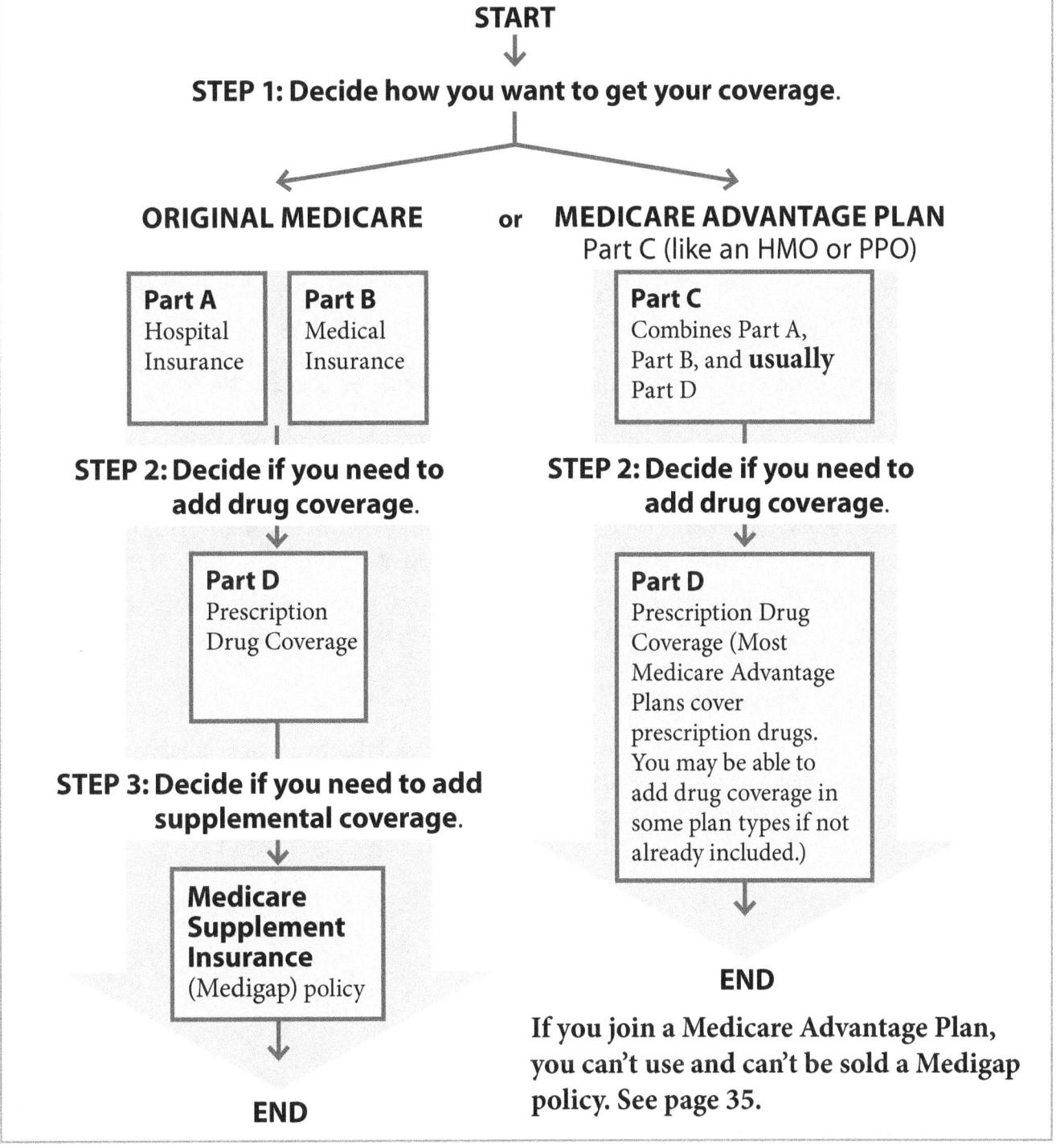

START

STEP 1: Decide how you want to get your coverage.

ORIGINAL MEDICARE or **MEDICARE ADVANTAGE PLAN**
Part C (like an HMO or PPO)

Part A
Hospital Insurance

Part B
Medical Insurance

Part C
Combines Part A, Part B, and **usually** Part D

STEP 2: Decide if you need to add drug coverage.

STEP 2: Decide if you need to add drug coverage.

Part D
Prescription Drug Coverage

Part D
Prescription Drug Coverage (Most Medicare Advantage Plans cover prescription drugs. You may be able to add drug coverage in some plan types if not already included.)

STEP 3: Decide if you need to add supplemental coverage.

Medicare Supplement Insurance (Medigap) policy

END

END

If you join a Medicare Advantage Plan, you can't use and can't be sold a Medigap policy. See page 35.

Medicare and the Health Insurance Marketplace

The Health Insurance Marketplace is a way for qualified individuals, families, and employees of small businesses to get health coverage. **Medicare isn't part of the Marketplace.**

Is Medicare coverage "minimum essential coverage?"

Minimum essential coverage is coverage that you need to have to meet the individual responsibility requirement under the Affordable Care Act.

As long as you have Medicare Part A (Hospital Insurance) coverage or are enrolled in a Medicare Advantage Plan, you have minimum essential coverage and you don't have to get any additional coverage.

If you only have Medicare Part B (Medical Insurance), you aren't considered to have minimum essential coverage. This means you may have to pay a fee for not having minimum essential coverage. You'd pay this fee when you file your federal income tax return.

Can I get a Marketplace plan instead of Medicare, or can I get a Marketplace plan in addition to Medicare?

Generally, no. In most cases, it's against the law for someone who knows you have Medicare to sell you a Marketplace plan, because that would duplicate your coverage. However, if you're employed and your employer offers employer-based coverage through the Marketplace, you may be eligible to get that type of coverage.

Note: The Marketplace doesn't offer Medicare Supplement Insurance (Medigap) policies, Medicare Advantage Plans, or Medicare drug plans (Part D).

For more information

Remember, this guide is about Medigap policies. To learn more about Medicare, visit Medicare.gov, look at your "Medicare & You" handbook, or call 1-800-MEDICARE (1-800-633-4227). TTY users should call 1-877-486-2048.

SECTION

2

Medigap Basics

What's a Medigap policy?

A Medigap policy is private health insurance that helps supplement Original Medicare. This means it helps pay some of the health care costs that Original Medicare doesn't cover (like copayments, coinsurance, and deductibles). These are "gaps" in Medicare coverage.

If you have Original Medicare and a Medigap policy, Medicare will pay its share of the Medicare-approved amounts for covered health care costs. Then your Medigap policy pays its share. A Medigap policy is different from a Medicare Advantage Plan (like an HMO or PPO) because those plans are ways to get Medicare benefits, while a Medigap policy only supplements the costs of your Original Medicare benefits.

Note: Medicare doesn't pay any of your costs for a Medigap policy.

All Medigap policies must follow federal and state laws designed to protect you, and policies must be clearly identified as "Medicare Supplement Insurance." Medigap insurance companies in most states can only sell you a "standardized" Medigap policy identified by letters A through N. Each standardized Medigap policy must offer the same basic benefits, no matter which insurance company sells it. **Cost is usually the only difference between Medigap policies with the same letter sold by different insurance companies.**

In Massachusetts, Minnesota, and Wisconsin, Medigap policies are standardized in a different way. See pages 42–44. In some states, you may be able to buy another type of Medigap policy called Medicare SELECT. Medicare SELECT plans are standardized plans that may require you to see certain providers and may cost less than other plans. See page 20.

What Medigap policies cover

The chart on page 11 gives you a quick look at the standardized Medigap Plans available. You'll need more details than this chart provides to compare and choose a policy. Call your State Health Insurance Assistance Program (SHIP) for help. See pages 47–48 for your state's phone number.

Notes:

- Insurance companies selling Medigap policies are required to make Plan A available. If they offer any other Medigap policy, they must also offer either Plan C or Plan F. Not all types of Medigap policies may be available in your state. See pages 42–44 if you live in **Massachusetts**, **Minnesota**, or **Wisconsin**.

- Plans D and G effective on or **after** June 1, 2010, **have different benefits** than Plans D or G bought **before** June 1, 2010.

- Plans E, H, I, and J are **no longer sold**, but, if you already have one, you can generally keep it.

This chart shows basic information about the different benefits that Medigap policies cover. If a percentage appears, the Medigap plan covers that percentage of the benefit, and you must pay the rest.

Benefits	Medicare Supplement Insurance (Medigap) Plans									
	A	B	C	D	F*	G	K	L	M	N
Medicare Part A coinsurance and hospital costs (up to an additional 365 days after Medicare benefits are used)	100%	100%	100%	100%	100%	100%	100%	100%	100%	100%
Medicare Part B coinsurance or copayment	100%	100%	100%	100%	100%	100%	50%	75%	100%	100% ***
Blood (first 3 pints)	100%	100%	100%	100%	100%	100%	50%	75%	100%	100%
Part A hospice care coinsurance or copayment	100%	100%	100%	100%	100%	100%	50%	75%	100%	100%
Skilled nursing facility care coinsurance			100%	100%	100%	100%	50%	75%	100%	100%
Part A deductible		100%	100%	100%	100%	100%	50%	75%	50%	100%
Part B deductible			100%		100%					
Part B excess charges					100%	100%				
Foreign travel emergency (up to plan limits)			80%	80%	80%	80%			80%	80%
Out-of-pocket limit in 2016**							$4,960	$2,480		

* Plan F is also offered as a high-deductible plan by some insurance companies in some states. If you choose this option, this means you must pay for Medicare-covered costs (coinsurance, copayments, deductibles) up to the deductible amount of $2,180 in 2016 before your policy pays anything.

**For Plans K and L, after you meet your out-of-pocket yearly limit and your yearly Part B deductible ($166 in 2016), the Medigap plan pays 100% of covered services for the rest of the calendar year.

*** Plan N pays 100% of the Part B coinsurance, except for a copayment of up to $20 for some office visits and up to a $50 copayment for emergency room visits that don't result in an inpatient admission.

What Medigap policies don't cover

Generally, Medigap policies don't cover long-term care (like care in a nursing home), vision or dental care, hearing aids, eyeglasses, or private-duty nursing.

Types of coverage that are NOT Medigap policies

- Medicare Advantage Plans (Part C), like an HMO, PPO, or Private Fee-for-Service Plan
- Medicare Prescription Drug Plans (Part D)
- Medicaid
- Employer or union plans, including the Federal Employees Health Benefits Program (FEHBP)
- TRICARE
- Veterans' benefits
- Long-term care insurance policies
- Indian Health Service, Tribal, and Urban Indian Health plans
- Qualified Health Plans sold in the Health Insurance Marketplace

What types of Medigap policies can insurance companies sell?

In most cases, Medigap insurance companies can sell you only a "standardized" Medigap policy. All Medigap policies must have specific benefits, so you can compare them easily. If you live in Massachusetts, Minnesota, or Wisconsin, see pages 42–44.

Words in blue are defined on pages 49–50.

Insurance companies that sell Medigap policies don't have to offer every Medigap plan. However, they must offer Plan A if they offer any Medigap policy. If they offer any plan in addition to Plan A, they must also offer Plan C or Plan F. Each insurance company decides which Medigap plan it wants to sell, although state laws might affect which ones they offer.

In some cases, an insurance company must sell you a Medigap policy, even if you have health problems. Here are certain times that you're guaranteed the right to buy a Medigap policy:

- When you're in your Medigap Open Enrollment Period. See pages 14–15.
- If you have a guaranteed issue right. See pages 21–23.

You may be able to buy a Medigap policy at other times, but the insurance company can deny you a Medigap policy based on your health. Also, in some cases it may be illegal for the insurance company to sell you a Medigap policy (like if you already have Medicaid or a Medicare Advantage Plan).

What do I need to know if I want to buy a Medigap policy?

- You must have Medicare Part A (Hospital Insurance) and Medicare Part B (Medical Insurance) to buy a Medigap policy.

- If you have a Medicare Advantage Plan (like an HMO or PPO) but are planning to return to Original Medicare, you can apply for a Medigap policy before your coverage ends. The Medigap insurer can sell it to you as long as you're leaving the Plan. Ask that the new Medigap policy start when your Medicare Advantage Plan enrollment ends, so you'll have continuous coverage.

- You pay the private insurance company a premium for your Medigap policy in addition to the monthly Part B premium you pay to Medicare.

- A Medigap policy only covers one person. If you and your spouse both want Medigap coverage, **you each will have to buy separate Medigap policies**.

- When you have your Medigap Open Enrollment Period, you can buy a Medigap policy from any insurance company that's licensed in your state.

- If you want to buy a Medigap policy, see page 11 for an overview of the basic benefits covered by different Medigap policies to review the benefit choices. Then, follow the "**Steps to Buying a Medigap Policy**" on pages 25–30.

- If you want to drop your Medigap policy, write your insurance company to cancel the policy and confirm it's cancelled. Your agent can't cancel the policy for you.

- Any standardized Medigap policy is guaranteed renewable even if you have health problems. This means the insurance company can't cancel your Medigap policy as long as you pay the premium.

- Different insurance companies may charge different premiums for the same exact policy. As you shop for a policy, be sure you're comparing the same policy (for example, compare Plan A from one company with Plan A from another company).

- Some states may have laws that may give you additional protections.

What do I need to know if I want to buy a Medigap policy? (continued)

- Although some Medigap policies sold in the past covered prescription drugs, Medigap policies sold after January 1, 2006, aren't allowed to include prescription drug coverage.

- If you want prescription drug coverage, you can join a Medicare Prescription Drug Plan (Part D) offered by private companies approved by Medicare. See pages 6–7.

To learn about Medicare prescription drug coverage, visit Medicare.gov, or call 1-800-MEDICARE (1-800-633-4227). TTY users should call 1-877-486-2048.

When's the best time to buy a Medigap policy?

The best time to buy a Medigap policy is during your Medigap Open Enrollment Period. This period lasts for 6 months and begins on the first day of the month in which you're both 65 or older and enrolled in Medicare Part B. Some states have additional Open Enrollment Periods including those for people under 65. During this period, an insurance company can't use medical underwriting. This means the insurance company can't do any of these because of your health problems:

- Refuse to sell you any Medigap policy it offers

- Charge you more for a Medigap policy than they charge someone with no health problems

- Make you wait for coverage to start (except as explained below)

Words in blue are defined on pages 49–50.

While the insurance company can't make you wait for your coverage to start, it may be able to make you wait for coverage related to a pre-existing condition. A pre-existing condition is a health problem you have before the date a new insurance policy starts. In some cases, the Medigap insurance company can refuse to cover your out-of-pocket costs for these pre-existing health problems for up to 6 months. This is called a "pre-existing condition waiting period." After 6 months, the Medigap policy will cover the pre-existing condition.

When's the best time to buy a Medigap policy? (continued)

Coverage for a pre-existing condition can only be excluded if the condition was treated or diagnosed within 6 months before the coverage starts under the Medigap policy. This is called the "look-back period." After the 6-month pre-existing condition waiting period, the Medigap policy will cover the condition that was excluded. Remember, for Medicare-covered services, Original Medicare will still cover the condition, even if the Medigap policy won't, but you're responsible for the Medicare coinsurance or copayment.

Creditable coverage

If you have a pre-existing condition, you buy a Medigap policy during your Medigap Open Enrollment Period, and you're replacing certain kinds of health coverage that count as "creditable coverage," it's possible to avoid or shorten waiting periods for pre-existing conditions. Prior creditable coverage is generally any other health coverage you recently had before applying for a Medigap policy. If you have had at least 6 months of continuous prior creditable coverage, the Medigap insurance company can't make you wait before it covers your pre-existing conditions.

There are many types of health care coverage that may count as creditable coverage for Medigap policies, but they'll only count if you didn't have a break in coverage for more than 63 days.

Your Medigap insurance company can tell you if your previous coverage will count as creditable coverage for this purpose. You can also call your State Health Insurance Assistance Program. See pages 47–48.

If you buy a Medigap policy when you have a guaranteed issue right (also called "Medigap protection"), the insurance company can't use a pre-existing condition waiting period. See pages 21–23 for more information about guaranteed issue rights.

Note: If you're under 65 and have Medicare because of a disability or End-Stage Renal Disease (ESRD), you might not be able to buy the Medigap policy you want, or any Medigap policy, until you turn 65. Federal law doesn't require insurance companies to sell Medigap policies to people under 65. However, some states require Medigap insurance companies to sell you a Medigap policy, even if you're under 65. See page 39 for more information.

Why is it important to buy a Medigap policy when I'm first eligible?

When you're first eligible, you have the right to buy any Medigap policy offered in your state. In addition, you generally will get better prices and more choices among policies. It's very important to understand your Medigap Open Enrollment Period. Medigap insurance companies are generally allowed to use medical underwriting to decide whether to accept your application and how much to charge you for the Medigap policy. However, if you apply during your Medigap Open Enrollment Period, you can buy any Medigap policy the company sells, even if you have health problems, for the same price as people with good health. If you apply for Medigap coverage **after** your Open Enrollment Period, there's no guarantee that an insurance company will sell you a Medigap policy if you don't meet the medical underwriting requirements, **unless** you're eligible because of one of the limited situations listed on pages 22–23.

It's also important to understand that your Medigap rights may depend on when you choose to enroll in Medicare Part B. If you're 65 or older, your Medigap Open Enrollment Period begins when you enroll in Part B and it can't be changed or repeated. In most cases, it makes sense to enroll in Part B and purchase a Medigap policy when you're first eligible for Medicare, because you might otherwise have to pay a Part B late enrollment penalty and you might miss your Medigap Open Enrollment Period. However, there are exceptions if you have employer coverage.

Employer coverage

Words in blue are defined on pages 49–50.

If you have group health coverage through an employer or union, because either you or your spouse is currently working, you may want to wait to enroll in Part B. This is because benefits based on current employment often provide coverage similar to Part B, so you would be paying for Part B before you need it, and your Medigap Open Enrollment Period might expire before a Medigap policy would be useful. When the employer coverage ends, you'll get a chance to enroll in Part B without a late enrollment penalty which means your Medigap Open Enrollment Period will start when you're ready to take advantage of it. If you enrolled in Part B while you still had employer coverage, your Medigap Open Enrollment Period would start, and unless you bought a Medigap policy before you needed it, you would miss your Medigap Open Enrollment Period entirely. If you or your spouse is still working and you have coverage through an employer, contact your employer or union benefits administrator to find out how your insurance works with Medicare. See page 24 for more information.

How do insurance companies set prices for Medigap policies?

Each insurance company decides how it'll set the price, or premium, for its Medigap policies. It's important to ask how an insurance company prices its policies. The way they set the price affects how much you pay now and in the future. Medigap policies can be priced or "rated" in 3 ways:

1. Community-rated (also called "no-age-rated")

2. Issue-age-rated (also called "entry-age-rated")

3. Attained-age-rated

Each of these ways of pricing Medigap policies is described in the chart on the next page. The examples show how your age affects your premiums, and why it's important to look at how much the Medigap policy will cost you now and in the future. The amounts in the examples aren't actual costs. Other factors like where you live, medical underwriting, and discounts can also affect the amount of your premium.

How do insurance companies set prices for Medigap policies? (continued)

Type of pricing	How it's priced	What this pricing may mean for you	Examples
Community-rated (also called "no-age-rated")	Generally the same premium is charged to everyone who has the Medigap policy, regardless of age or gender.	Your premium isn't based on your age. Premiums may go up because of inflation and other factors but not because of your age.	Mr. Smith is 65. He buys a Medigap policy and pays a $165 monthly premium.
			Mrs. Perez is 72. She buys the same Medigap policy as Mr. Smith. She also pays a $165 monthly premium because, with this type of Medigap pricing, everyone pays the same price regardless of age.
Issue-age-rated (also called "entry age-rated")	The premium is based on the age you are when you buy (are "issued") the Medigap policy.	Premiums are lower for people who buy at a younger age and won't change as you get older. Premiums may go up because of inflation and other factors but not because of your age.	Mr. Han is 65. He buys a Medigap policy and pays a $145 monthly premium.
			Mrs. Wright is 72. She buys the same Medigap policy as Mr. Han. Since she is older when she buys it, her monthly premium is $175.
Attained-age-rated	The premium is based on your current age (the age you've "attained"), so your premium goes up as you get older.	Premiums are low for younger buyers but go up as you get older. They may be the least expensive at first, but they can eventually become the most expensive. Premiums may also go up because of inflation and other factors.	Mrs. Anderson is 65. She buys a Medigap policy and pays a $120 monthly premium. Her premium will go up each year: • At 66, her premium goes up to $126. • At 67, her premium goes up to $132. • At 72, her premium goes up to $165.
			Mr. Dodd is 72. He buys the same Medigap policy as Mrs. Anderson. He pays a $165 monthly premium. His premium is higher than Mrs. Anderson's because it's based on his current age. Mr. Dodd's premium will go up each year: • At 73, his premium goes up to $171. • At 74, his premium goes up to $177.

Comparing Medigap costs

As discussed on the previous pages, the cost of Medigap policies can vary widely. **There can be big differences in the premiums that different insurance companies charge for exactly the same coverage**. As you shop for a Medigap policy, be sure to compare the same type of Medigap policy, and consider the type of pricing used. See pages 17–18. For example, compare a Plan C from one insurance company with a Plan C from another insurance company. Although this guide **can't** give actual costs of Medigap policies, you can get this information by calling insurance companies or your State Health Insurance Assistance Program. See pages 47–48.

You can also find out which insurance companies sell Medigap policies in your area by visiting Medicare.gov.

The cost of your Medigap policy may also depend on whether the insurance company:

- Offers discounts (like discounts for women, non-smokers, or people who are married; discounts for paying yearly; discounts for paying your premiums using electronic funds transfer; or discounts for multiple policies).

- Uses medical underwriting, or applies a different premium when you don't have a guaranteed issue right or aren't in a Medigap Open Enrollment Period.

- Sells Medicare SELECT policies that may require you to use certain providers. If you buy this type of Medigap policy, your premium may be less. See page 20.

- Offers a "high-deductible option" for Plan F. If you buy Plan F with a high-deductible option, you must pay the first $2,180 of deductibles, copayments, and coinsurance (in 2016) not paid by Medicare before the Medigap policy pays anything. You must also pay a separate deductible ($250 per year) for foreign travel emergency services.

If you bought your Medigap Plan J before January 1, 2006, and it still covers prescription drugs, you would also pay a separate deductible ($250 per year) for prescription drugs covered by the Medigap policy. And, if you have a Plan J with a high deductible option, you must also pay a $2,180 deductible (in 2016) before the policy pays anything for medical benefits.

What's Medicare SELECT?

Medicare SELECT is a type of Medigap policy sold in some states that requires you to use hospitals and, in some cases, doctors within its network to be eligible for full insurance benefits (except in an emergency). Medicare SELECT can be any of the standardized Medigap plans (see page 11). These policies generally cost less than other Medigap policies. However, if you don't use a Medicare SELECT hospital or doctor for non-emergency services, you'll have to pay some or all of what Medicare doesn't pay. Medicare will pay its share of approved charges no matter which hospital or doctor you choose.

How does Medigap help pay my Medicare Part B bills?

In most Medigap policies, when you sign the Medigap insurance contract you agree to have the Medigap insurance company get your Medicare Part B claim information directly from Medicare, and then they pay the doctor directly whatever amount is owed under your policy. Some Medigap insurance companies also provide this service for Medicare Part A claims.

If your Medigap insurance company **doesn't** provide this service, ask your doctors if they participate in Medicare. Participating providers have signed an arrangement to accept assignment for all Medicare-covered services. If your doctor participates, the Medigap insurance company is required to pay the doctor directly if you request. If your doctor doesn't participate but still accepts Medicare, you may be asked to pay the coinsurance amount at the time of service. In these cases, your Medigap insurance company will pay you directly according to policy limits.

If you have any questions about Medigap claim filing, call 1-800-MEDICARE (1-800-633-4227). TTY users should call 1-877-486-2048.

Your Right to Buy a Medigap Policy

What are guaranteed issue rights?

As explained on pages 14–16, the best time to buy a Medigap policy is during your Medigap Open Enrollment Period, when you have the right to buy any Medigap policy offered in your state. However, even if you aren't in your Medigap Open Enrollment Period, there are several situations in which you may still have a guaranteed right to buy a Medigap policy.

Guaranteed issue rights are rights you have in certain situations when insurance companies must offer you certain Medigap policies. In these situations, an insurance company must:

- Sell you a Medigap policy
- Cover all your pre-existing health conditions
- Can't charge you more for a Medigap policy regardless of past or present health problems

If you live in Massachusetts, Minnesota, or Wisconsin, you have guaranteed issue rights to buy a Medigap policy, but the Medigap policies are different. See pages 42–44 for your Medigap policy choices.

When do I have guaranteed issue rights?

In most cases, you have a guaranteed issue right when you have certain types of other health care coverage that changes in some way, like when you lose the other health care coverage. In other cases, you have a "trial right" to try a Medicare Advantage Plan and still buy a Medigap policy if you change your mind. For information on trial rights, see page 23.

This chart describes the situations, under federal law, that give you a right to buy a policy, the kind of policy you can buy, and when you can or must apply for it. States may provide additional Medigap guaranteed issue rights.

You have a guaranteed issue right if...	You have the right to buy...	You can/must apply for a Medigap policy...
You're in a Medicare Advantage Plan (like an HMO or PPO), and your plan is leaving Medicare or stops giving care in your area, or you move out of the plan's service area.	Medigap Plan A, B, C, F, K, or L that's sold in your state by any insurance company. You only have this right if you switch to Original Medicare rather than join another Medicare Advantage Plan.	As early as 60 calendar days before the date your health care coverage will end, but no later than 63 calendar days after your health care coverage ends. Medigap coverage can't start until your Medicare Advantage Plan coverage ends.
You have Original Medicare and an employer group health plan (including retiree or COBRA coverage) or union coverage that pays after Medicare pays and that plan is ending. **Note:** In this situation, you may have additional rights under state law.	Medigap Plan A, B, C, F, K, or L that's sold in your state by any insurance company. If you have COBRA coverage, you can either buy a Medigap policy right away or wait until the COBRA coverage ends.	No later than 63 calendar days after the latest of these 3 dates: 1. Date the coverage ends 2. Date on the notice you get telling you that coverage is ending (if you get one) 3. Date on a claim denial, if this is the only way you know that your coverage ended
You have Original Medicare and a Medicare SELECT policy. You move out of the Medicare SELECT policy's service area. Call the Medicare SELECT insurer for more information about your options.	Medigap Plan A, B, C, F, K, or L that's sold by any insurance company in your state or the state you're moving to.	As early as 60 calendar days before the date your Medicare SELECT coverage will end, but no later than 63 calendar days after your Medicare SELECT coverage ends.

This chart describes the situations, under federal law, that give you a right to buy a policy, the kind of policy you can buy, and when you can or must apply for it. States may provide additional Medigap guaranteed issue rights. (continued)

You have a guaranteed issue right if...	You have the right to buy...	You can/must apply for a Medigap policy...
(**Trial right**) You joined a Medicare Advantage Plan (like an HMO or PPO) or Programs of All-inclusive Care for the Elderly (PACE) when you were first eligible for Medicare Part A at 65, and within the first year of joining, you decide you want to switch to Original Medicare.	Any Medigap policy that's sold in your state by any insurance company.	As early as 60 calendar days before the date your coverage will end, but no later than 63 calendar days after your coverage ends. **Note:** Your rights may last for an extra 12 months under certain circumstances.
(**Trial right**) You dropped a Medigap policy to join a Medicare Advantage Plan (or to switch to a Medicare SELECT policy) for the first time, you've been in the plan less than a year, and you want to switch back.	The Medigap policy you had before you joined the Medicare Advantage Plan or Medicare SELECT policy, if the same insurance company you had before still sells it. If your former Medigap policy **isn't** available, you can buy Medigap Plan A, B, C, F, K, or L that's sold in your state by any insurance company.	As early as 60 calendar days before the date your coverage will end, but no later than 63 calendar days after your coverage ends. **Note:** Your rights may last for an extra 12 months under certain circumstances.
Your Medigap insurance company goes bankrupt and you lose your coverage, or your Medigap policy coverage otherwise ends through no fault of your own.	Medigap Plan A, B, C, F, K, or L that's sold in your state by any insurance company.	No later than 63 calendar days from the date your coverage ends.
You leave a Medicare Advantage Plan or drop a Medigap policy because the company hasn't followed the rules, or it misled you.	Medigap Plan A, B, C, F, K, or L that's sold in your state by any insurance company.	No later than 63 calendar days from the date your coverage ends.

Can I buy a Medigap policy if I lose my health care coverage?

Yes, you may be able to buy a Medigap policy. Because you may have a guaranteed issue right to buy a Medigap policy, make sure you keep these:

- A copy of any letters, notices, emails, and/or claim denials that have your name on them as proof of your coverage being terminated.

- The postmarked envelope these papers come in as proof of when it was mailed.

You may need to send a copy of some or all of these papers with your Medigap application to prove you have a guaranteed issue right.

If you have a Medicare Advantage Plan (like an HMO or PPO) but you're planning to return to Original Medicare, you can apply for a Medigap policy before your coverage ends. The Medigap insurer can sell it to you as long as you're leaving the plan. Ask that the new policy take effect when your Medicare Advantage enrollment ends, so you'll have continuous coverage.

For more information

If you have any questions or want to learn about any additional Medigap rights in your state, you can:

- Call your State Health Insurance Assistance Program to make sure that you qualify for these guaranteed issue rights. See pages 47–48.

- Call your State Insurance Department if you're denied Medigap coverage in any of these situations. See pages 47–48.

Important: The guaranteed issue rights in this section are from federal law. These rights are for both Medigap and Medicare SELECT policies. Many states provide additional Medigap rights.

There may be times when more than one of the situations in the chart on pages 22–23 applies to you. When this happens, you can choose the guaranteed issue right that gives you the best choice.

Some of the situations listed include loss of coverage under Programs of All-inclusive Care for the Elderly (PACE). PACE combines medical, social, and long-term care services, and prescription drug coverage for frail people. To be eligible for PACE, you must meet certain conditions. PACE may be available in states that have chosen it as an optional Medicaid benefit. If you have Medicaid, an insurance company can sell you a Medigap policy **only** in certain situations. For more information about PACE, visit Medicare.gov, or call 1-800-MEDICARE (1-800-633-4227). TTY users should call 1-877-486-2048.

Steps to Buying a Medigap Policy

Step-by-step guide to buying a Medigap policy

Buying a **Medigap policy** is an important decision. Only you can decide if a Medigap policy is the way for you to supplement Original Medicare coverage and which Medigap policy to choose. Shop carefully. Compare available Medigap policies to see which one meets your needs. As you shop for a Medigap policy, keep in mind that different insurance companies may charge different amounts for exactly the same Medigap policy, and not all insurance companies offer all of the Medigap policies.

Below is a step-by-step guide to help you buy a Medigap policy. If you live in Massachusetts, Minnesota, or Wisconsin, see pages 42–44.

STEP 1: Decide which benefits you want, then decide which of the standardized Medigap policies meet your needs.

STEP 2: Find out which insurance companies sell Medigap policies in your state.

STEP 3: Call the insurance companies that sell the Medigap policies you're interested in and compare costs.

STEP 4: Buy the Medigap policy.

STEP 1: Decide which benefits you want, then decide which of the Medigap policy meets your needs.

You should think about your current and future health care needs when deciding which benefits you want because you might not be able to switch Medigap policies later. Decide which benefits you need, and select the Medigap policy that will work best for you. The chart on page 11 provides an overview of Medigap benefits.

STEP 2: Find out which insurance companies sell Medigap policies in your state.

To find out which insurance companies sell Medigap policies in your state:

- Call your State Health Insurance Assistance Program. See pages 47–48. Ask if they have a "Medigap rate comparison shopping guide" for your state. This guide usually lists companies that sell Medigap policies in your state and their costs.

- Call your State Insurance Department. See pages 47–48.

- Visit Medicare.gov/find-a-plan:

  This website will help you find information on all your health plan options, including the Medigap policies in your area. You can also get information on:

  ✔ How to contact the insurance companies that sell Medigap policies in your state.

  ✔ What each Medigap policy covers.

  ✔ How insurance companies decide what to charge you for a Medigap policy premium.

Words in blue are defined on pages 49–50.

If you don't have a computer, your local library or senior center may be able to help you look at this information. You can also call 1-800-MEDICARE (1-800-633-4227). A customer service representative will help you get information on all your health plan options including the Medigap policies in your area. TTY users should call 1-877-486-2048.

STEP 2: (continued)

Since costs can vary between companies, you should plan to call more than one insurance company that sells Medigap policies in your state. Before you call, check the companies to be sure they're honest and reliable by using one of these resources:

- Call your State Insurance Department. Ask if they keep a record of complaints against insurance companies that can be shared with you. When deciding which Medigap policy is right for you, consider these complaints, if any.

- Call your State Health Insurance Assistance Program. These programs can give you help with choosing a Medigap policy at no cost to you.

- Go to your local public library for help with:
  - Getting information on an insurance company's financial strength from independent rating services like weissratings.com, A.M. Best, and Standard & Poor's.
  - Looking at information about the insurance company online.

- Talk to someone you trust, like a family member, your insurance agent, or a friend who has a Medigap policy from the same Medigap insurance company.

STEP 3: **Call the insurance companies that sell the Medigap policies you're interested in and compare costs.**

Before you call any insurance companies, figure out if you're in your Medigap Open Enrollment Period or if you have a guaranteed issue right. Read pages 14–15 and 22–23 carefully. If you have questions, call your State Health Insurance Assistance Program. See pages 47–48. This chart can help you keep track of the information you get.

Ask each insurance company...	Company 1	Company 2
"Are you licensed in ___?" (Say the name of your state.) **Note:** If the answer is NO, STOP here, and try another company.		
"Do you sell Medigap Plan ___?" (Say the letter of the Medigap Plan you're interested in.) **Note:** Insurance companies usually offer some, but not all, Medigap policies. Make sure the company sells the plan you want. Also, if you're interested in a Medicare SELECT or high-deductible Medigap policy, tell them.		
"Do you use medical underwriting for this Medigap policy?" **Note:** If the answer is NO, go to step 4 on page 30. If the answer is YES, but you know you're in your Medigap Open Enrollment Period or have a guaranteed issue right to buy that Medigap policy, go to step 4. Otherwise, you can ask, "Can you tell me whether I'm likely to qualify for the Medigap policy?"		
"Do you have a waiting period for pre-existing conditions?" **Note:** If the answer is YES, ask how long the waiting period is and write it in the box.		
"Do you price this Medigap policy by using community-rating, issue-age-rating, or attained-age-rating?" See page 18. **Note:** Circle the one that applies for that insurance company.	Community Issue-age Attained-age	Community Issue-age Attained-age
"I'm ___ years old. What would my premium be under this Medigap policy?" **Note:** If it's attained-age, ask, "How frequently does the premium increase due to my age?"		
"Has the premium for this Medigap policy increased in the last 3 years due to inflation or other reasons?" **Note:** If the answer is YES, ask how much it has increased, and write it in the box.		
"Do you offer any discounts or additional benefits?" See page 19.		

STEP 3: (continued)

Watch out for illegal practices.

It's illegal for anyone to:

- Pressure you into buying a Medigap policy, or lie to or mislead you to switch from one company or policy to another.

- Sell you a second Medigap policy when they know that you already have one, unless you tell the insurance company in writing that you plan to cancel your existing Medigap policy.

- Sell you a Medigap policy if they know you have Medicaid, except in certain situations.

- Sell you a Medigap policy if they know you're in a Medicare Advantage Plan (like an HMO or PPO) unless your coverage under the Medicare Advantage Plan will end before the effective date of the Medigap policy.

- Claim that a Medigap policy is a part of Medicare or any other federal program. Medigap is private health insurance.

- Claim that a Medicare Advantage Plan is a Medigap policy.

- Sell you a Medigap policy that can't legally be sold in your state. Check with your State Insurance Department (see pages 47–48) to make sure that the Medigap policy you're interested in can be sold in your state.

- Misuse the names, letters, or symbols of the U.S. Department of Health & Human Services (HHS), Social Security Administration (SSA), Centers for Medicare & Medicaid Services (CMS), or any of their various programs like Medicare. (For example, they can't suggest the Medigap policy has been approved or recommended by the federal government.)

- Claim to be a Medicare representative if they work for a Medigap insurance company.

- Sell you a Medicare Advantage Plan when you say you want to stay in Original Medicare and buy a Medigap policy. A Medicare Advantage Plan isn't the same as Original Medicare. See page 5. If you enroll in a Medicare Advantage Plan, you can't use a Medigap policy.

If you believe that a federal law has been broken, call the Inspector General's hotline at 1-800-HHS-TIPS (1-800-447-8477). TTY users should call 1-800-377-4950. Your State Insurance Department can help you with other insurance-related problems.

STEP 4: Buy the Medigap policy.

Once you decide on the insurance company and the Medigap policy you want, you should apply. The insurance company must give you a clearly worded summary of your Medigap policy. Read it carefully. If you don't understand it, ask questions. Remember these when you buy your Medigap policy:

- **Filling out your application.** Fill out the application carefully and completely, including medical questions. The answers you give will determine your eligibility for an Open Enrollment Period or guaranteed issue rights. If the insurance agent fills out the application, make sure it's correct. If you buy a Medigap policy during your Medigap Open Enrollment Period or provide evidence that you're entitled to a guaranteed issue right, the insurance company can't use any medical answers you give to deny you a Medigap policy or change the price. The insurance company can't ask you any questions about your family history or require you to take a genetic test.

- **Paying for your Medigap policy.** You can pay for your Medigap policy by check, money order, or bank draft. Make it payable to the insurance company, not the agent. If buying from an agent, get a receipt with the insurance company's name, address, and phone number for your records. Some companies may offer electronic funds transfer.

- **Starting your Medigap policy.** Ask for your Medigap policy to become effective when you want coverage to start. Generally, Medigap policies begin the first of the month after you apply. If, for any reason, the insurance company won't give you the effective date for the month you want, call your State Insurance Department. See pages 47–48.

  Note: If you already have a Medigap policy, ask for your new Medigap policy to become effective when your old Medigap policy coverage ends.

- **Getting your Medigap policy.** If you don't get your Medigap policy in 30 days, call your insurance company. If you don't get your Medigap policy in 60 days, call your State Insurance Department.

If you already have a Medigap policy, it's illegal for an insurance company to sell you a second policy unless you tell them in writing that you'll cancel the first Medigap policy. However, don't cancel your old Medigap policy until the new one is in place, and you decide to keep it. See pages 29 and 32.

SECTION 5

If You Already Have a Medigap Policy

You should read this section if any of these situations apply to you:

- You're thinking about switching to a different Medigap policy. See pages 32–35.

- You're losing your Medigap coverage. See page 36.

- You have a Medigap policy with Medicare prescription drug coverage. See pages 36–38.

If you just want a refresher about Medigap insurance, turn to page 11.

Switching Medigap policies

If you're satisfied with your current Medigap policy's cost, coverage, and customer service, you don't need to do anything. If you're thinking about switching to a new Medigap policy, see below and pages 33–35 to answer some common questions about switching Medigap policies.

Can I switch to a different Medigap policy?

In most cases, you won't have a right under federal law to switch Medigap policies, unless you're within your 6-month Medigap Open Enrollment Period or are eligible under a specific circumstance for guaranteed issue rights. But, if your state has more generous requirements, or the insurance company is willing to sell you a Medigap policy, make sure you compare benefits and premiums before switching. If you bought your Medigap policy before 2010, it may offer coverage that isn't available in a newer Medigap policy. On the other hand, Medigap policies bought before 1992 might not be guaranteed renewable and might have bigger premium increases than newer, standardized Medigap policies currently being sold.

If you decide to switch, don't cancel your first Medigap policy until you've decided to keep the second Medigap policy. On the application for the new Medigap policy, you'll have to promise that you'll cancel your first Medigap policy. You have 30 days to decide if you want to keep the new Medigap policy. This is called your "free look period." The 30-day free look period starts when you get your new Medigap policy. You'll need to pay both premiums for one month.

Words in blue are defined on pages 49–50.

Switching Medigap policies (continued)

Do I have to switch Medigap policies if I have a Medigap policy that's no longer sold?

No. But you can't have more than one Medigap policy, so if you buy a new Medigap policy, you have to give up your old policy (except for your 30-day "free look period," described on page 32). Once you cancel the policy, you can't get it back.

Do I have to wait a certain length of time after I buy my first Medigap policy before I can switch to a different Medigap policy?

No. If you've had your old Medigap policy for less than 6 months, the Medigap insurance company may be able to make you wait up to 6 months for coverage of a pre-existing condition. However, if your old Medigap policy had the same benefits, and you had it for 6 months or more, the new insurance company can't exclude your pre-existing condition. If you've had your Medigap policy less than 6 months, the number of months you've had your current Medigap policy must be subtracted from the time you must wait before your new Medigap policy covers your pre-existing condition.

If the new Medigap policy has a benefit that isn't in your current Medigap policy, you may still have to wait up to 6 months before that benefit will be covered, regardless of how long you've had your current Medigap policy.

If you've had your current Medigap policy longer than 6 months and want to replace it with a new one with the same benefits and the insurance company agrees to issue the new policy, they can't write pre-existing conditions, waiting periods, elimination periods, or probationary periods into the replacement policy.

Switching Medigap policies (continued)

Why would I want to switch to a different Medigap policy?

Some reasons for switching may include:

- You're paying for benefits you don't need.

- You need more benefits than you needed before.

- Your current Medigap policy has the right benefits, but you want to change your insurance company.

- Your current Medigap policy has the right benefits, but you want to find a policy that's less expensive.

It's important to compare the benefits in your current Medigap policy to the benefits listed on page 11. If you live in Massachusetts, Minnesota, or Wisconsin, see pages 42–44. To help you compare benefits and decide which Medigap policy you want, follow the "**Steps to Buying a Medigap Policy**" in Section 4. If you decide to change insurance companies, you can call the new insurance company and arrange to apply for your new Medigap policy. If your application is accepted, call your current insurance company, and ask to have your coverage end. The insurance company can tell you how to submit a request to end your coverage.

As discussed on page 32, you should have your old Medigap policy coverage end **after** you have the new Medigap policy for 30 days. Remember, this is your 30-day free look period. You'll need to pay both premiums for one month.

Switching Medigap policies (continued)

Can I keep my current Medigap policy (or Medicare SELECT policy) or switch to a different Medigap policy if I move out-of-state?

In general, you can keep your current Medigap policy regardless of where you live as long as you still have Original Medicare. If you want to switch to a different Medigap policy, you'll have to check with your current or the new insurance company to see if they'll offer you a different Medigap policy.

You may have to pay more for your new Medigap policy and answer some medical questions if you're buying a Medigap policy outside of your Medigap Open Enrollment Period. See pages 14–16.

If you have a Medicare SELECT policy and you move out of the policy's area, you can:

• Buy a standardized Medigap policy from your current Medigap policy insurance company that offers the same or fewer benefits than your current Medicare SELECT policy. If you've had your Medicare SELECT policy for more than 6 months, you won't have to answer any medical questions.

• Use your guaranteed issue right to buy any Plan A, B, C, F, K, or L that's sold in most states by any insurance company.

Your state may provide additional Medigap rights. Call your State Health Insurance Assistance Program or State Department of Insurance for more information. See pages 47–78 for their phone numbers.

What happens to my Medigap policy if I join a Medicare Advantage Plan?

Words in blue are defined on pages 49–50.

Medigap policies can't work with Medicare Advantage Plans. If you decide to keep your Medigap policy, you'll have to pay your Medigap policy premium, but the Medigap policy can't pay any deductibles, copayments, coinsurance, or premiums under a Medicare Advantage Plan. So, if you join a Medicare Advantage Plan, you may want to drop your Medigap policy. Contact your Medigap insurance company to find out how to disenroll. However, if you leave the Medicare Advantage Plan you might not be able to get the same Medigap policy back, or in some cases, any Medigap policy unless you have a "trial right." See page 23. Your rights to buy a Medigap policy may vary by state. You always have a legal right to keep the Medigap policy after you join a Medicare Advantage Plan. However, because you have a Medicare Advantage Plan, the Medigap policy would no longer provide benefits that supplement Medicare.

Losing Medigap coverage

Can my Medigap insurance company drop me?

If you bought your Medigap policy **after 1992**, in most cases the Medigap insurance company can't drop you because the Medigap policy is guaranteed renewable. This means your insurance company can't drop you unless one of these happens:

- You stop paying your premium.
- You weren't truthful on the Medigap policy application.
- The insurance company becomes bankrupt or insolvent.

If you bought your Medigap policy **before 1992**, it might not be guaranteed renewable. This means the Medigap insurance company can refuse to renew the Medigap policy, as long as it gets the state's approval to cancel your Medigap policy. However, if this does happen, you have the right to buy another Medigap policy. See the guaranteed issue right on page 23.

Medigap policies and Medicare prescription drug coverage

If you bought a Medigap policy **before** January 1, 2006, and it has coverage for prescription drugs, see below and page 37.

Medicare offers prescription drug coverage (Part D) for everyone with Medicare. If you have a Medigap policy with prescription drug coverage, that means you chose not to join a Medicare Prescription Drug Plan when you were first eligible. However, you can still join a Medicare drug plan. Your situation may have changed in ways that make a Medicare drug plan fit your needs better than the prescription drug coverage in your Medigap policy. It's a good idea to review your coverage each fall, because you can join a Medicare drug plan between October 15–December 7. Your new coverage will begin on January 1.

Medigap policies and Medicare prescription drug coverage (continued)

Why would I change my mind and join a Medicare drug plan?

In a Medicare Prescription Drug Plan, you may have to pay a monthly premium, but Medicare pays a large part of the cost. There's no maximum yearly amount as with Medigap prescription drug benefits in old Plans H, I, and J (these plans are no longer sold). However, a Medicare drug plan might only cover certain prescription drugs (on its "formulary" or "drug list"). It's important that you check whether your current prescription drugs are on the Medicare drug plan's list of covered prescription drugs before you join.

If your Medigap premium or your prescription drug needs were very low when you had your first chance to join a Medicare drug plan, your Medigap prescription drug coverage may have met your needs. However, if your Medigap premium or the amount of prescription drugs you use has increased recently, a Medicare drug plan might now be a better choice for you.

Will I have to pay a late enrollment penalty if I join a Medicare drug plan now?

If you qualify for Extra Help, you won't pay a late enrollment penalty. If you don't qualify for Extra Help, it will depend on whether your Medigap policy includes "creditable prescription drug coverage." This means that the Medigap policy's drug coverage pays, on average, at least as much as Medicare's standard prescription drug coverage.

If your Medigap policy's drug coverage **isn't** creditable coverage, and you join a Medicare drug plan now, you'll probably pay a higher premium (a penalty added to your monthly premium) than if you had joined when you were first eligible. Each month that you wait to join a Medicare drug plan will make your late enrollment penalty higher. Your Medigap carrier must send you a notice each year telling you if the prescription drug coverage in your Medigap policy is creditable. You should keep these notices in case you decide later to join a Medicare drug plan. You should also consider that your prescription drug needs could increase as you get older.

Will I have to pay a late enrollment penalty if I join a Medicare drug plan now? (continued)

If your Medigap policy includes creditable prescription drug coverage and you decide to join a Medicare Prescription Drug Plan, you won't have to pay a late enrollment penalty as long as you don't go 63 or more days in a row without creditable prescription drug coverage. So, don't drop your Medigap policy **before** you join the Medicare drug plan and the coverage starts. You can only join a Medicare drug plan between October 15–December 7 unless you lose your Medigap policy (for example, if it isn't guaranteed renewable, and your company cancels it). In that case, you may be able to join a Medicare drug plan at the time you lose your Medigap policy.

Can I join a Medicare drug plan and have a Medigap policy with prescription drug coverage?

No. If your Medigap policy covers prescription drugs, you must tell your Medigap insurance company if you join a Medicare drug plan so it can remove the prescription drug coverage from your Medigap policy and adjust your premium. Once the drug coverage is removed, you can't get that coverage back even though you didn't change Medigap policies.

What if I decide to drop my entire Medigap policy (not just the Medigap prescription drug coverage) and join a Medicare Advantage Plan that offers prescription drug coverage?

You need to be careful about the timing because in general, you can only join a Medicare Prescription Drug Plan or Medicare Advantage Plan (like an HMO or PPO) during the Open Enrollment Period between October 15–December 7. If you join during an Open Enrollment Period, your coverage will begin on January 1 as long as the plan gets your enrollment request by December 7.

SECTION

Medigap Policies for People with a Disability or ESRD

Information for people under 65

Medigap policies for people under 65 and eligible for Medicare because of a disability or End-Stage Renal Disease (ESRD)

You may have Medicare before turning 65 due to a disability or ESRD (permanent kidney failure requiring dialysis or a kidney transplant).

If you're a person with Medicare under 65 and have a disability or ESRD, you might not be able to buy the Medigap policy you want, or any Medigap policy, until you turn 65. Federal law generally doesn't require insurance companies to sell Medigap policies to people under 65. However, some states require Medigap insurance companies to sell you a Medigap policy, even if you're under 65. These states are listed on the next page.

Important: This section provides information on the minimum federal standards. For your state requirements, call your State Health Insurance Assistance Program. See pages 47–48.

Medigap policies for people under 65 and eligible for Medicare because of a disability or End-Stage Renal Disease (ESRD) (continued)

At the time of printing this guide, these states required insurance companies to offer at least one kind of Medigap policy to people with Medicare under 65:

• California	• Maine	• North Carolina
• Colorado	• Maryland	• Oklahoma
• Connecticut	• Massachusetts	• Oregon
• Delaware	• Michigan	• Pennsylvania
• Florida	• Minnesota	• South Dakota
• Georgia	• Mississippi	• Tennessee
• Hawaii	• Missouri	• Texas
• Illinois	• Montana	• Vermont
• Kansas	• New Hampshire	• Wisconsin
• Kentucky	• New Jersey	
• Louisiana	• New York	

Note: Some states provide these rights to all people with Medicare under 65, while others only extend them to people eligible for Medicare because of disability or only to people with ESRD. Check with your State Insurance Department about what rights you might have under state law.

Even if your state isn't on the list above, some insurance companies may voluntarily sell Medigap policies to people under 65, although they'll probably cost you more than Medigap policies sold to people over 65, and they can probably use medical underwriting. Also, some of the federal guarantee rights are available to people with Medicare under 65, see pages 21-24. Check with your State Insurance Department about what additional rights you might have under state law.

Remember, if you're already enrolled in Medicare Part B, you'll get a Medigap Open Enrollment Period when you turn 65. You'll probably have a wider choice of Medigap policies and be able to get a lower premium at that time. During the Medigap Open Enrollment Period, insurance companies can't refuse to sell you any Medigap policy due to a disability or other health problem, or charge you a higher premium (based on health status) than they charge other people who are 65.

Because Medicare (Part A and/or Part B) is creditable coverage, if you had Medicare for more than 6 months before you turned 65, you may not have a pre-existing condition waiting period. For more information about the Medigap Open Enrollment Period and pre-existing conditions, see pages 16–17. If you have questions, call your State Health Insurance Assistance Program. See pages 47–48.

Words in blue are defined on pages 49–50.

Medigap Coverage in Massachusetts, Minnesota, and Wisconsin

Massachusetts—Chart of standardized Medigap policies

Massachusetts benefits

- **Inpatient hospital care:** covers the Medicare Part A coinsurance plus coverage for 365 additional days after Medicare coverage ends
- **Medical costs:** covers the Medicare Part B coinsurance (generally 20% of the Medicare-approved amount)
- **Blood:** covers the first 3 pints of blood each year
- Part A hospice coinsurance or copayment

The check marks in this chart mean the benefit is covered.

Medigap benefits	Core plan	Supplement 1 Plan
Basic benefits	✓	✓
Part A: inpatient hospital deductible		✓
Part A: skilled nursing facility (SNF) coinsurance		✓
Part B: deductible		✓
Foreign travel emergency		✓
Inpatient days in mental health hospitals	60 days per calendar year	120 days per benefit year
State-mandated benefits (annual Pap tests and mammograms. Check your plan for other state-mandated benefits.)	✓	✓

For more information on these Medigap policies, visit Medicare.gov/find-a-plan, or call your State Insurance Department. See pages 47–48.

Minnesota—Chart of standardized Medigap policies

Minnesota benefits

- **Inpatient hospital care:** covers the Part A coinsurance
- **Medical costs:** covers the Part B coinsurance (generally 20% of the Medicare-approved amount)
- **Blood:** covers the first 3 pints of blood each year
- Part A hospice and respite cost sharing
- Parts A and B home health services and supplies cost sharing

The check marks in this chart mean the benefit is covered.

Medigap benefits	Basic plan	Extended basic plan
Basic benefits	✓	✓
Part A: inpatient hospital deductible		✓
Part A: skilled nursing facility (SNF) coinsurance	✓ (Provides 100 days of SNF care)	✓ (Provides 120 days of SNF care)
Part B: deductible		✓
Foreign travel emergency	80%	80%*
Outpatient mental health	20%	20%
Usual and customary fees		80%*
Medicare-covered preventive care	✓	✓
Physical therapy	20%	20%
Coverage while in a foreign country		80%*
State-mandated benefits (diabetic equipment and supplies, routine cancer screening, reconstructive surgery, and immunizations)	✓	✓

Mandatory riders

Insurance companies can offer 4 additional riders that can be added to a basic plan. You may choose any one or all of these riders to design a Medigap policy that meets your needs:

1. Part A: inpatient hospital deductible
2. Part B: deductible
3. Usual and customary fees
4. Non-medicare preventive care

* Pays 100% after you spend $1,000 in out-of-pocket costs for a calendar year.

Minnesota versions of Medigap Plans K, L, M, N, and high-deductible F are available.

Important: The basic and extended basic benefits are available when you enroll in Part B, regardless of age or health problems. If you are under 65, return to work and drop Part B to elect your employer's health plan, you'll get a 6-month Medigap Open Enrollment Period after you retire from that employer when you can elect Part B again.

Wisconsin — Chart of standardized Medigap policies

Wisconsin benefits

- **Inpatient hospital care:** covers the Part A coinsurance
- **Medical costs:** covers the Part B coinsurance (generally 20% of the Medicare-approved amount)
- **Blood:** covers the first 3 pints of blood each year
- Part A hospice coinsurance or copayment

The check marks in this chart mean the benefit is covered.

Medigap benefits	Basic plan	Optional riders
Basic benefits	✓	Insurance companies are allowed to offer these 7 additional riders to a Medigap policy:
Part A: skilled nursing facility (SNF) coinsurance	✓	1. Part A deductible
Inpatient mental health coverage	175 days per lifetime in addition to Medicare's benefit	2. Additional home health care (365 visits including those paid by Medicare)
Home health care	40 visits per year in addition to those paid by Medicare	3. Part B deductible 4. Part B excess charges 5. Foreign travel emergency
State-mandated benefits	✓	6. 50% Part A deductible 7. Part B copayment or coinsurance

For more information on these Medigap policies, visit Medicare.gov/find-a-plan or call your State Insurance Department. See pages 47–48.

Plans known as "50% and 25% cost-sharing plans" are available. These plans are similar to standardized Plans K (50%) and L (25%). A high-deductible plan ($2,180 deductible for 2016) is also available.

SECTION

8

For More Information

Where to get more information

On pages 47–48, you'll find phone numbers for your State Health Insurance Assistance Program (SHIP) and State Insurance Department.

- Call your SHIP for help with:
    - Buying a Medigap policy or long-term care insurance.
    - Dealing with payment denials or appeals.
    - Medicare rights and protections.
    - Choosing a Medicare plan.
    - Deciding whether to suspend your Medigap policy.
    - Questions about Medicare bills.

- Call your State Insurance Department if you have questions about the Medigap policies sold in your area or any insurance-related problems.

How to get help with Medicare and Medigap questions

If you have questions about Medicare, Medigap, or need updated phone numbers for the contacts listed on pages 47–48:

Visit Medicare.gov:

- For Medigap policies in your area, visit Medicare.gov/find-a-plan.
- For updated phone numbers, visit Medicare.gov/contacts.

Call 1-800-MEDICARE (1-800-633-4227):

Customer service representatives are available 24 hours a day, 7 days a week. TTY users should call 1-877-486-2048. If you need help in a language other than English or Spanish, let the customer service representative know the language.

State Health Insurance Assistance Program and State Insurance Department

State	State Health Insurance Assistance Program	State Insurance Department
Alabama	1-800-243-5463	1-800-433-3966
Alaska	1-800-478-6065	1-800-467-8725
American Samoa	Not available	1-684-633-4116
Arizona	1-800-432-4040	1-800-325-2548
Arkansas	1-800-224-6330	1-800-224-6330
California	1-800-434-0222	1-800-927-4357
Colorado	1-888-696-7213	1-800-930-3745
Connecticut	1-800-994-9422	1-800-203-3447
Delaware	1-800-336-9500	1-800-282-8611
Florida	1-800-963-5337	1-877-693-5236
Georgia	1-866-552-4464	1-800-656-2298
Guam	1-671-735-7421	1-671-635-1835
Hawaii	1-888-875-9229	1-808-586-2790
Idaho	1-800-247-4422	1-800-721-4422
Illinois	1-217-524-6911	1-888-473-4858
Indiana	1-800-452-4800	1-800-622-4461
Iowa	1-800-351-4664	1-877-955-1212
Kansas	1-800-860-5260	1-800-432-2484
Kentucky	1-877-293-7447	1-800-595-6053
Louisiana	1-800-259-5300	1-800-259-5301
Maine	1-877-353-3771	1-800-300-5000
Maryland	1-800-243-3425	1-800-492-6116
Massachusetts	1-800-243-4636	1-877-563-4467
Michigan	1-800-803-7174	1-877-999-6442
Minnesota	1-800-333-2433	1-800-657-3602
Mississippi	1-800-948-3090	1-800-562-2957
Missouri	1-800-390-3330	1-800-726-7390
Montana	1-800-551-3191	1-800-332-6148
Nebraska	1-800-234-7119	1-800-234-7119

State	State Health Insurance Assistance Program	State Insurance Department
Nevada	1-800-307-4444	1-800-992-0900
New Hampshire	1-866-634-9412	1-800-852-3416
New Jersey	1-800-792-8820	1-800-446-7467
New Mexico	1-800-432-2080	1-888-727-5772
New York	1-800-701-0501	1-800-342-3736
North Carolina	1-800-443-9354	1-800-546-5664
North Dakota	1-800-247-0560	1-800-247-0560
Northern Mariana Islands	Not available	1-670-664-3064
Ohio	1-800-686-1578	1-800-686-1526
Oklahoma	1-800-763-2828	1-800-522-0071
Oregon	1-800-722-4134	1-888-877-4894
Pennsylvania	1-800-783-7067	1-877-881-6388
Puerto Rico	1-877-725-4300	1-888-722-8686
Rhode Island	1-401-462-0510	1-401-462-9500
South Carolina	1-800-868-9095	1-803-737-6160
South Dakota	1-800-536-8197	1-605-773-3563
Tennessee	1-877-801-0044	1-800-342-4029
Texas	1-800-252-9240	1-800-252-3439
Utah	1-800-541-7735	1-800-439-3805
Vermont	1-800-642-5119	1-800-964-1784
Virgin Islands	1-340-772-7368 1-340-714-4354 (St. Thomas)	1-340-774-7166
Virginia	1-800-552-3402	1-877-310-6560
Washington	1-800-562-6900	1-800-562-6900
Washington D.C.	1-202-994-6272	1-202-727-8000
West Virginia	1-877-987-4463	1-888-879-9842
Wisconsin	1-800-242-1060	1-800-236-8517
Wyoming	1-800-856-4398	1-800-438-5768

Definitions

Where words in BLUE are defined

Assignment—An agreement by your doctor, provider, or supplier to be paid directly by Medicare, to accept the payment amount Medicare approves for the service, and not to bill you for any more than the Medicare deductible and coinsurance.

Coinsurance—An amount you may be required to pay as your share of the costs for services after you pay any deductibles. Coinsurance is usually a percentage (for example, 20%).

Copayment—An amount you may be required to pay as your share of the cost for a medical service or supply, like a doctor's visit, hospital outpatient visit, or a prescription. A copayment is usually a set amount, rather than a percentage. For example, you might pay $10 or $20 for a doctor's visit or prescription.

Deductible—The amount you must pay for health care or prescriptions, before Original Medicare, your prescription drug plan, or your other insurance begins to pay.

Excess charge—If you have Original Medicare, and the amount a doctor or other health care provider is legally permitted to charge is higher than the Medicare-approved amount, the difference is called the excess charge.

Guaranteed issue rights—Rights you have in certain situations when insurance companies are required by law to sell or offer you a Medigap policy. In these situations, an insurance company can't deny you a Medigap policy, or place conditions on a Medigap policy, such as exclusions for pre-existing conditions, and can't charge you more for a Medigap policy because of a past or present health problem.

Guaranteed renewable policy—An insurance policy that can't be terminated by the insurance company unless you make untrue statements to the insurance company, commit fraud, or don't pay your premiums. All Medigap policies issued since 1992 are guaranteed renewable.

Medicaid—A joint federal and state program that helps with medical costs for some people with limited income and resources. Medicaid programs vary from state to state, but most health care costs are covered if you qualify for both Medicare and Medicaid.

Medical underwriting—The process that an insurance company uses to decide, based on your medical history, whether or not to take your application for insurance, whether or not to add a waiting period for pre-existing conditions (if your state law allows it), and how much to charge you for that insurance.

Medicare Advantage Plan (Part C)—A type of Medicare health plan offered by a private company that contracts with Medicare to provide you with all your Medicare Part A and Part B benefits. Medicare Advantage Plans include Health Maintenance Organizations, Preferred Provider Organizations, Private Fee-for-Service Plans, Special Needs Plans, and Medicare Medical Savings Account Plans. If you're enrolled in a Medicare Advantage Plan, Medicare services are covered through the plan and aren't paid for under Original Medicare. Most Medicare Advantage Plans offer prescription drug coverage.

Medicare-approved amount—In Original Medicare, this is the amount a doctor or supplier that accepts assignment can be paid. It may be less than the actual amount a doctor or supplier charges. Medicare pays part of this amount and you're responsible for the difference.

Medicare prescription drug plan (Part D)—Part D adds prescription drug coverage to Original Medicare, some Medicare Cost Plans, some Medicare Private-Fee-for-Service Plans, and Medicare Medical Savings Account Plans. These plans are offered by insurance companies and other private companies approved by Medicare. Medicare Advantage Plans may also offer prescription drug coverage that follows the same rules as Medicare Prescription Drug Plans.

Medicare SELECT—A type of Medigap policy that may require you to use hospitals and, in some cases, doctors within its network to be eligible for full benefits.

Open Enrollment Period (Medigap)—A one-time-only, 6-month period when federal law allows you to buy any Medigap policy you want that's sold in your state. It starts in the first month that you're covered under Medicare Part B, **and** you're 65 or older. During this period, you can't be denied a Medigap policy or charged more due to past or present health problems. Some states may have additional Open Enrollment rights under state law.

Premium—The periodic payment to Medicare, an insurance company, or a health care plan for health care or prescription drug coverage.

State Health Insurance Assistance Program (SHIP)—A state program that gets money from the Federal government to give free local health insurance counseling to people with Medicare.

State Insurance Department—A state agency that regulates insurance and can provide information about Medigap policies and other private health insurance.

U.S. DEPARTMENT OF
HEALTH AND HUMAN SERVICES

Centers for Medicare & Medicaid Services
7500 Security Boulevard
Baltimore, Maryland 21244-1850

Official Business
Penalty for Private Use, $300

CMS Product No. 02110
Revised April 2016

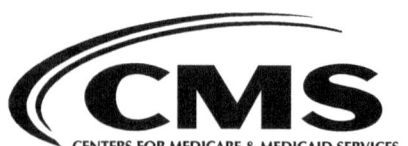

To get this publication in Braille, Spanish, or large print (English), visit Medicare.gov, or call 1-800-MEDICARE (1-800-633-4227). TTY users should call 1-877-486-2048.

¿Necesita una copia en español? Visite Medicare.gov en el sitio Web. Para saber si esta publicación esta impresa y disponible (en español), llame GRATIS al 1-800-MEDICARE (1-800-633-4227). Los usuarios de TTY deben llamar al 1-877-486-2048.

www.ingramcontent.com/pod-product-compliance
Lightning Source LLC
Chambersburg PA
CBHW081119280526
45787CB00007B/2906